HOW TO GET RID OF SHOULDER PAIN FAST

By

Mrs. Pain Free

TABLE OF CONTENTS

Dedication

This book is dedicated to all those who are experiencing shoulder pain in their life.

I dealt with pain for over six months and lost mobility from a simple muscle strain. I cannot take medicines due to physical sensitivities, so I had to find a natural way to get rid of my shoulder pain fast. Through much prayer and research, I found the solution that worked for me and I am sharing it with you in hopes it will get rid of your pain fast.

I do not guarantee this will work for you but it's worth a try. I do advise you to speak with your physician prior to trying the techniques mentioned in this book. Suggestions are not FDA approved and the reader accepts all responsibility for their actions regarding the information provided in this book.

Enjoy this journey with me…

Pain Story

Are you experiencing this now?

The groan was heartfelt and deep from her soul.

For the umpteenth time that day, Adele grabbed her shoulder, wincing in extreme pain. With every movement of her body, she felt the pain down to her core, bringing tears to her eyes. It was excruciating; she couldn't do anything with the shoulder since the pain began. It was like a thousand needles were in her muscles and joints, constantly tearing at her everywhere.

Now, she couldn't even do something as simple as shopping for groceries at the mall.

Adele had tried everything she could about the pain since it started. All her friends had advised various things and she had tried out every single suggestion. It was all to no avail; it was like some terrible monster had decided to make her shoulder its abode. She couldn't concentrate on her studies at the university anymore. Her part time job as a waitress was becoming too much to handle because she couldn't hold on to the trays without crying out. Thank goodness for her friend, Mary who was helping her with her shifts, she would have lost her job.

She couldn't even carry a handbag on her shoulder anymore. Now, she carried a clutch purse with her everywhere she went. The pain was disrupting her life, her work and everything she held dear.

Gingerly, Adele inched over to the shelf, trying to rake the needed groceries into her shopping cart.

"Ow! Ouch!" she screamed out loud this time around, grabbing her shoulder as the pain came back with vengeance.

She released her hold on the shopping cart and the packs of coffee pack fell to the floor. She couldn't even be bothered about the fallen items on the floor. The pain in her shoulder was killing her – it certainly felt like she was dying.

"Excuse me, miss, are you alright?"

Adele heard someone talking to her alright but she couldn't reply – not just yet. Her eyes were shut tightly – she didn't know if it was to hold back the mortifying tears of pain from flowing or to hold the pain in check. The pain began to recede but only a little and she breathed easier, her breaths coming up in short gasps.

This pain would be the death of her, it was certain.

"Miss?" the man called again.

Slowly, Adele opened her eyes to see a male attendant staring at her worriedly. He was a young man – he couldn't be a year or two older than her twenty two years – and he seemed genuinely worried for her. He had the air of a college student and she guessed he was working a part time job too. She tried to drum up a smile but it came out as a grimace.

"Yes, I am alright, thank you," she managed to grit out.

The pain was still there, hampering her usually bright smile and cordial relationship with people even strangers.

The attendant looked like he didn't believe her but he shrugged hesitantly and bent over to pick the packs of coffee off the floor. Adele slowly bent over to help him and immediately, the pain sliced through her skin again. This time, she couldn't hold back the tears of pain as two rapid drops slid down her cheeks.

She moaned out loud, holding her shoulders again and leaning against the shelf of groceries.

"Miss!" the attendant called in alarm, rushing over to her side.

Without another word, the attendant helped her to a sitting position on the floor, careful not to touch her left shoulder.

"You need to see a doctor about that shoulder, miss," the attendant said. "Did you bring a car? Should I call an ambulance for you?"

"Yes, I brought a car but no, no hospital," Adele murmured, shaking her head in agitated refusal.

She had been there and done that. She was not going to the hospital, no thank you!

"But you seem to be in serious pain, miss...?" the attendant said as he helped her up and outside the store.

Adele tried to control her breath as she realized that the attendant was asking for her name.

"Adele," she supplied hurriedly, "Adele Washington. You may call me Adele."

"Alright, Adele, you may call me Eric. You really need to get someone to see that shoulder right now," he said as they reached her beat-up Mercedes.

"I will be fine," she reassured the man. "It is just a little shoulder strain."

"That is not *just* a little shoulder strain," Eric gave her a level look. "I know a bit about strain, especially shoulder strains, and by the look of pain on your face some minutes ago, it hurts horribly."

Adele could not deny that so she simply kept quiet, massaging her shoulder with her fingers.

"Since you seem averse to seeing a doctor about that pain, if you don't mind, could I recommend some therapy for you?"

Adele snorted in as ladylike a manner as she could manage given the pain.

"I have tried everything, even Chinese therapy," she told him.

He raised a thick brow that suggested he felt she didn't know what she was saying and she was obliged to explain. "Yes, I saw some Chinese doctor and it wasn't your usual acupuncture he used on me. The man used some hard core massage that scared me to death. Believe me, the pain almost killed me but I bore it because the man assured me that the pain would be gone like it was never there. As you can see, he lied."

The bitterness was obvious in her voice – as it should be. She had tried everything from pain killers to massage and the Chinese remedy she just told Eric now. Now, she was resigned to fate, she wasn't going to use anything anymore. She had since restricted herself to relaxing massages and that was all. She was not going to try anything else before the pain ate her out of her entire savings and scholarship grants.

Eric seemed to be in thought before he said another word.

"What I have in mind isn't your usual Chinese therapy, it is some sort of new therapy that only a few people know about," Eric said softly.

"No, thank you," Adele replied immediately. She grabbed the steering wheel to let him know she wanted to leave now.

Eric eased away from her car only an inch.

"You know what I said about knowing a bit about shoulder strains?" Eric asked suddenly.

Adele nodded in exasperation. She was going to go now, she only needed a moment more so the pain could let her drive.

"You see, I used to have this shoulder pain too, the kind that felt like my shoulder was going to tear off like someone was holding some tiny needles to it."

Adele gasped. It was exactly how it felt when the pain started. "How did you get yours?" Eric asked.

"From trying to reach for a glass cup of water while on bed," she replied immediately, now interested in what he had to say.

She still found it funny that such a simple action could be the harbinger for such excruciating pain as she had been put to in the past month.

"And I bet you had no idea that the pain would last this long," Eric told her with a smile. "I got mine from sitting at a desk too long. You know that shoulder strain is quite the rage these days, right? Many people keep the pain for so long hoping it would go away on its own but it doesn't."

"How did you heal yours?" Adele asked interestedly.

"That is the new therapy I was telling you about," Eric smiled. "A friend of mine introduced me to this doctor…"

Slowly, Adele got her hands off the wheel. She listened as Eric filled her in about this new therapy that had helped him. If all Eric was telling her was true, then all hope was not lost for her. Impulsively, she decided that she was going to give this therapy one last attempt. She was too young to spend the rest of her life with a perpetual shoulder pain.

"How can I get started with this therapy?"

That Shoulder Pain!

Okay, so it's only a shoulder pain, there's nothing much to it and pretty soon, it's going to disappear unannounced just the way it came. Well, you may be right – and then, you just might not.

A lot of people fall into the category of ignoring pains in their body system – they go on and say, "As long as I can still go about my normal everyday activities, then, I am fine!"

So, Adele goes right on to ignore the stiffness in her shoulder, Eric simply stretches his triceps and biceps once or twice at his desk to get rid of the persistent soreness at his upper back and Mrs. Whoever simply takes painkillers to dull those aches that send sharp needle-like pricks from her shoulders all the way to her neck.

If it were that simple, the statistics wouldn't have so much to say about shoulder pain – and so many people wouldn't be in so much trouble and pain for it.

So, before you go right on to relegate that telltale sign of shoulder pain in the category of 'nothing serious to worry about', here are a few things you might want to know about shoulder pain.

The Shoulders, What They Are

Basically, we all know the shoulder as a perfect synchrony of the long bone of the upper arm bone, the collarbone and the shoulder blades nicely wrapped up by cartilages and muscles. All in all, they form a ball and socket joint that we all call the shoulder joint. Now, this joint is by no means irrelevant in the everyday movement and activities of the human.

With its large range of motion which includes moving the entire shoulder back and forth and the movement of the arms in all allowable directions, the shoulder joint is the most mobile joint in the body yet! Its freedom of expression tells on our posture, bearing, gait, body position and other physical activities such as swimming, walking, etc.

Now, imagine an unwieldy shoulder joint. There you have it, undesirable right?

That Pain in my Shoulders, What does it really mean?

Pain in the shoulders is a common complaint in the healthcare industry. Contrary to popular opinion, it not only affects the old but also all age groups only with a higher percentage in the older age range.

Shoulder pains can be derived from a range of physical activities ranging from seemingly harmless ones as those involved at work such as typing or sitting at a desk too long, to a session of tennis on the field, sudden movement which puts pressure on the shoulder and monotonous actions that weren't even supposed to be any bother at all.

Diseases related to the liver, heart and spinal cord are also known to have caused serious shoulder pains. And oh, you don't have to worry; shoulder pain has nothing to do with genetics. But then with age, you might just have to worry about the pain because well, at old age, tissues and muscles deteriorate and those girding up the shoulders are no different.

Sometimes, it's both shoulders and other times, it's only one shoulder with this pain. In some cases, the pain only comes once in a while but in other cases, it is persistent and hinders day to day activities. While other pains can be ignored, some shoulder pains can only scream, "Here I am!"

Shoulder pain can be as worse as giving you sleepless nights, restless days, mood swings, loss of concentration, referred pains to other body parts, disrupted days and permanent discomfort in the region of pain. It can aggravate other medical conditions if not duly treated and may be responsible for chest and neck pains if left unattended for long.

What Causes My Shoulder Pain?

As mentioned above, the causes of shoulder pains range from a number of common and uncommon sources. To cut off the medical jargon, here are a few that you probably can reckon with right away:

1. Injury to the neck – or other nearby regions – which extends to the shoulder

2. Inflammation of the tendons surrounding the shoulders

3. Shoulder dislocation

4. Repetitive posture over a long period of time; e.g, sitting at a desk

5. Sudden stiffening of shoulder

6. Arthritis

7. Over use of shoulder muscles as in during exercises in the gym

8. Old age

9. Related diseases

While a series of the above-mentioned causes might be the reason your shoulder hurts, there may be so many others you just might not pay attention to. As an example, a patent without any history of shoulder pain once reached out for a glass of water, felt her shoulder muscles cramp up and there on, she began to nurse serious pains in her shoulders. Yes, it actually could be something as mundane as reaching for a glass.

There you have it, found anything familiar? Well, not to panic; not every sudden jerk or motion causes shoulder pain so there should be no paranoia involved here. With the causes listed above, you can better take note of any pain in your shoulders so you could easily diagnose such pains and report them immediately.

Just so you know – shoulder pain left too long is simply a no-no.

So, as Adele wanted to know, what therapy can heal my shoulder pain fast?

<u>THE SOLUTION FOR ME</u>

First, think about when the shoulder pain started. Was it an injury or just something that built up slowly over time?

If it was an injury, then healing time must be allowed, sometimes up to a year depending on how bad the injury was.

For myself, I had an injury and after six months, my shoulder pain was getting worse. My shoulder injury was most likely a tear in my rotator cuff or some tendons and muscles. I did not get a formal doctor diagnosis as I could not use drugs due to reactions from them.

So off I went through the natural healing process for pain. Acupuncture plus Chinese herbs worked for a few weeks but then the pain started getting worse again. Deep tissue massages were too painful to tolerate.

What could I do? Go to youtube online and start looking up exercises that might heal my shoulder. I found two different programs that worked with FAST results!

Program 1 - (I am not liable in any way regarding these exercises, please check with your doctor prior to trying them as you are responsible for your own body)

1. Neck exercises that stretched the spine, shoulder and neck muscles that were compressed and causing the pain.

    A. Gently pull up the hair on the top of your head to get in an upright position. Once in this position, slowly slide your chin back (you can lightly use a finger on your chin to push it back - maybe 1/4 inch...do not force it back... just do this until you cannot go back any further), hold for 3 seconds and release. Do this 10 times every hour for the first day.

B. You wake up on the second day, do you still have pain? If so, do the same straightening as in "A" but this time, gently tilt your head back and look left and right (slightly turning your head) without forcing, like watching a tennis match. Do this 3 times each way and release. Do this exercise 10 times every hour for the second day.

C. You wake up on the third day, do you still have pain? If so, (this was the one that solved my problem), then pull up your hair to get in an upright position, push your chin back and tilt your head to the each side - is one side easier to do then the other? If so, tilt your head to that side and hold for three seconds, release and do this ten times every hour. If you cannot tell which is tighter, then do it both directions.

Program 2 - (I am not liable in any way regarding these exercises, please check with your doctor prior to trying them as you are responsible for your own body)

1. Program 1 got rid of my pain fast but I also wanted a way to heal my shoulder instead of just relieving my pain. So, this is what I did.

2. Check your body for any tightness in any area head to toe. For example, raise one arm close to your ear and see how far back it will go. Now do the same with the other arm. Does one arm go back further than the other? If so, you are out of alignment.

3. Following the example above, exercise the best range of motion arm. Go to youtube online and search on total motion release for your arm or shoulder.   I think what you find, you will be pleasantly surprised. And yes, I am not going to give you all my secrets but if you do the suggested research online, you will find the answers and you will become pain free possibly without drugs or even surgery. I avoided drugs and surgery.

4. Consider prayer. It has been scientifically proven that relaxation and meditation relieves stress which causes neck, shoulder and back pains. I had two people lay hands on my shoulder and prayed for healing. I felt a warm sensation, about a couple of hours later, that came from the inside out.   For example, when one uses a heating pad, the heat goes from the pad to the area of treatment.   What happened to me was the heat went from inside of the treatment area out for about two hours, while I was relaxing for sleep. I give all honor to our God in Heaven for the healing of my shoulder. Just know, a little prayer goes a long way!

Enjoy your healing journey and I pray this path is a blessing to you in your life!

***Again, know that any exercises you do from the recommendations in this book are your responsibility. We are not liable in any way. Please check with your doctor or therapist or both prior to doing any exercise. ***